Table of contents

Introduction

What is Bariatric diet?

How does bariatric diet works?

Foods to consume

Recipes and procedures

Conclusion

Introduction

The term bariatrics was coined around 1965, from the Greek root bar- ("weight" as in barometer), suffix -iatr ("treatment," as in pediatrics), and suffix -ic ("pertaining to"). The field encompasses dieting, exercise and behavioral therapy approaches to weight loss, as well as pharmacotherapy and surgery. The term is also used in the medical field as somewhat of a euphemism to refer to people of larger sizes without regard to their participation in any treatment specific to weight loss, such as medical supply catalogs featuring larger hospital gowns and hospital beds referred to as "bariatric".

Bariatric patients

Being overweight or obese are both rising medical problems. There are many detrimental health effects of obesity: Individuals with a BMI (Body Mass Index) exceeding a healthy range have a much greater risk of medical issues. These include heart disease, diabetes mellitus, many types of cancer, asthma, obstructive sleep apnea, and chronic musculoskeletal problems.

There is also a focus on the correlation between obesity and mortality.

Overweight and obese people, including children, may find it difficult to lose weight on their own. It is common for dieters to have tried fad diets only to find that they gain weight, or return to their original weight, after ceasing the diet. Some improvement in patient psychological health is noted after bariatric surgery. 51% of bariatric surgery candidates report a history of mental illness, specifically depression, as well as being prescribed at least one psychotropic medication at the time of their surgery candidacy.

Methods of treatment

Although diet, exercise, behavior therapy and anti-obesity drugs are first-line treatment, medical therapy for severe obesity has limited short-term success and very poor long-term success. Weight loss surgery generally results in greater weight loss than conventional treatment, and leads to improvements in quality of life and obesity related diseases such as hypertension and diabetes mellitus. A meta-analysis of 174772 participants published in The Lancet in 2021 found that bariatric surgery was associated with 59% and 30% reduction in all-cause mortality among obese adults with or without type 2 diabetes respectively. This meta-analysis also found that median life-expectancy was 9.3 years longer for obese adults with diabetes who received bariatric surgery as compared to routine (non-surgical) care, whereas the life expectancy gain was 5.1 years longer for obese adults without diabetes.

The combination of approaches used may be tailored to each patient.[18] Bariatric treatments in youth must be considered with great caution and with other conditions that may not have to be considered in adults.

Bariatric Diet Recipes

As part of the lifestyle changes needed following bariatric surgery, individuals will need to make changes towards a healthy lifestyle, especially in regard to food and diet.

This usually means choosing more nutritionally dense food and eating smaller portions. While this can be overwhelming, it is critical for maintaining long-term success.

To help make this process a bit easier, a collection of 18 of the best bariatric diet recipes are listed below.

1. Skinny Meatloaf Muffins with Barbecue Sauce

Who can resist muffins, especially ones full of meat? This is one of those bariatric diet recipes that brings together your favorite flavors of meatloaf in easy-to-control portion servings.

Ground turkey and whole wheat breadcrumbs are used, making this a great choice for anyone looking for a healthier version of traditional meatloaf.

Tip: Do not be afraid to experiment with different flavors of BBQ sauce.

2. Chipotle Chicken Fajita Bowls

In a time crunch and need to get dinner on the table fast? With some high protein recipes, bariatric patients can do just that and still stick to their diet.

This is one of them! It is low in carbs and calories but full of flavor. These bowls can also be customized to suit varying tastes and diets.

Cheese can be added to the mix, the cauliflower swapped out for rice or beans, or it can even be made into a salad.

3. Healthy Low Carb Breakfast Burritos

Who says you can't enjoy bacon and cheese while preparing gastric bypass recipes? These easy breakfast burritos allow you to do just that!

They are low in carbs and high in protein and come in perfect portion-controlled sizes.

This recipe can be used as a base and any of your favorite toppings can be added. It is freezer-friendly, so make a double batch to ensure you always have something healthy to grab in the morning.

Tip: To keep the carb count down on this, make sure that you are using low-carb tortillas.

4. Keto Sour Cream Chicken Enchiladas

Looking for weight loss surgery recipes that still allow you to enjoy your favorite Mexican dishes?

You can, with this easy recipe. It gives traditional enchiladas a keto-friendly makeover.

The secret is replacing the tortillas with cauliflower rice. The result is a delicious tasting, low-carb meal that can be ready in under 30 minutes.

5. Low Carb Keto Chicken Enchiladas

Can enchiladas still be enjoyed while preparing bariatric diet recipes? Absolutely! This recipe lets you do just that by using low-carb tortillas.

Simply cook the chicken and veggies, place them in the tortillas, top them with cheese and sauce, and put them in the oven to bake. In no time, you will have a dish full of Mexican flavor.

Serve this alongside a simple salad or cauliflower rice for a complete meal.

6. Lemon Garlic Butter Salmon Baked in Foil

This is one of those high protein recipes bariatric patients will savor, as will the rest of the family.

The best part? It comes together in under 20 minutes, using basic pantry staples. Season the salmon, seal it in a foil packet and bake it for 10-15 minutes.

In the time it takes you to prepare a salad to go along with it, the salmon will be done and a restaurant-quality dinner on the table.

7. Strawberry Lemon

Need a refreshing summer treat that you don't feel guilty about? With these healthy strawberry and lemon popsicles that meet all the requirements for gastric bypass recipes, you can still indulge in your favorite summer treat.

Blend together lemon juice, water, sugar, and strawberries, place the mixture in popsicle molds, and put them in the freezer.

The hardest part of this recipe is waiting for the popsicles to freeze!

Tip: Swap out the strawberries for whatever fruit is in season.

8. Vegan Lentil, Haricot Bean & Chickpea Soup

Searching for high protein recipes bariatric patients that are vegetarians can enjoy?

This simple dish is just what you are looking for! Lentils, chickpeas, and beans are the star of this soup that is full of protein and will keep you feeling full for hours.

Tip: If you like your soup on the spicier side, try adding some chili powder for a hit of heat.

9. Easy Cajun Cauliflower Rice

Who doesn't love a healthy one-pan meal that is low in carbs? This is one of those weight loss surgery recipes that checks off all the boxes!

This easy cauliflower rice dish is full of flavor, requires only six ingredients, and can be prepared in under 20 minutes.

It is filling enough to serve as a main meal and goes great with a salad or veggies.

10. No-Carb Cloud Bread

Have you heard of cloud bread yet? It is the bread that has no carbs, making it one of the best choices for any weight loss surgery recipes that require bread. Only four basic ingredients are needed to make cloud bread and the process is fairly simple.

Tip: Make sure to take the time to beat the egg whites until they are completely stiff, as that is key to making the bread fluffy and soft.

11. Keto Spaghetti Squash Au Gratin

Are you looking for a way to incorporate a wider variety of veggies into your menu planning for bariatric diet recipes?

This spaghetti squash recipe is a delicious and healthy choice, especially in the fall when the squash is in season.

By using spaghetti squash, it puts a low-carb spin on traditional potatoes au gratin. This recipe is easy to make and will make the perfect side dish for any meal.

12. Instant Pot White Chicken Chili Verde

How can you go wrong with chili? Especially if it requires little prep, tastes delicious, and is healthy for you!

With this recipe all you have to do is prep a few veggies, combine them with chicken, seasonings, and a bit of broth and water.

Let them cook and do their thing and then using an immersion blender, blend the soup to your preferred consistency.

While the original version of this recipe uses an InstaPot, it could also be prepared as one of those bariatric slow cooker recipes.

13. Golden red & orange bell pepper soup

Wondering if it possible to make a creamy soup, without using any dairy? With these bariatric diet recipes, you can!

The secret is using sweet potatoes in place of the dairy.

Simply cook onions, carrots, and celery until tender, add in some bell peppers, sweet potatoes, and broth, and let simmer until everything is tender.

Once the soup has cooled a bit, use an immersion blender to blend the soup to your desired consistency.

The final result is a vibrant colored creamy soup, that packs a powerful nutritional punch.

14. Whole30 BLT Chicken Salad

In search of a healthy alternative to a traditional BLT? This is one of those gastric bypass recipes that puts a healthy twist on an old favorite.

All you have to do is cook your bacon and chicken and then mix them together with mayonnaise, green onions, pepper, and cherry tomatoes. Serve this keto-friendly salad in lettuce cups or just on its own.

Tip: To save time and make this recipe even easier, use a rotisserie chicken from the grocery store.

15. Powder mug cake recipe

Fudgy gooey brownies that are healthy and full of protein? Yes, please! Not many weight loss surgery recipes will satisfy your sweet tooth, like this one for keto brownies does.

The secret ingredient that makes this magic possible is protein powder. As an added bonus, this recipe is for a single serving which helps to keep your portion control in check.

Tip: To make your brownies even more fudgy and moist, cook them for slightly less time than listed.

16. Bacon cheeseburger cauliflower casserole

Need a sure-fire dish to impress any crowd? With this recipe, ground beef, cheese, and bacon are layered over a cauliflower crust and topped with sauce to create a delicious casserole that would rival any hamburger.

This is one of those bariatric diet recipes that will become a family favorite and might even replace a traditional hamburger.

17. The Best Keto Meatloaf Minis With Low Carb Ketchup

Looking for gastric by-pass recipes that can be prepped ahead of time and are pre-portioned?? Stop searching, these easy mini meatloaves are a perfect idea.

They have a shortlist of ingredients, come together quickly, and are keto-friendly.

Do yourself a favor and make a double batch of these, serve some immediate and keep the rest in the freezer.

18. Low carb pizza casserole

Love pizza but not all the calories and carbs that come along with it?

This is one of those weight loss surgery ideas that let you indulge in the taste of pizza, without the guilt.

Sausages, mushrooms, green peppers, and cauliflower are mixed together and layered with cheese and sauce to make a pizza-like casserole that will win over even the pickiest eaters.

WHAT IS IN A BREAKFAST BURRITO

There is no right or wrong way to make a breakfast burrito. As long as there are eggs and low carb tortillas, the rest is up to you. Here are ingredients you can add in your burrito:

- scrambled eggs

- cheese

- bacon, ham, sausage

- peppers

- onions

- spinach

- tomatoes

- avocado

- mushrooms

- chives

I love being creative with my burritos, but with four kids, I prefer a simple, hearty breakfast, which is why I chose to make this burrito recipe with just a few staple ingredients; Eggs, bacon, and cheese.

HOW TO MAKE LOW CARB BREAKFAST BURRITOS

, these burrito wraps are not 100% keto-friendly because many who follow a strict keto diet avoid wheat; however, they ARE low carb! If you avoid grains on keto, this would be the perfect recipe to try for a "cheat day" without having carb-overload.

I used a brand that has just 16 grams of carbs with 11 grams of fiber, making them only 5 grams of net carbs. (Check out the brand in my recipe below.) Some tortillas can contain up to 26 grams of carbs, so compare labels at the grocery store if you can't find the brand I used.

To make this easy burrito, get your ingredients prepared first. You will need to pre-cook your eggs and bacon. Also, have your tortillas ready to go.

You can choose any tortilla you like but look for the low carb variety if you're sticking to a semi-keto friendly diet. They have so many tortilla options in the store, so find one you like best that suits your dietary needs.

Next, take your scrambled egg mixture, shredded cheese, and crumbled bacon and add to the center of each tortilla. You want to be generous with your filling but not too generous, so you can't roll your burritos.

Tip: In this recipe, I used sharp cheddar cheese and white cheddar cheese, but feel free to use any other cheese that you prefer.

Roll each burrito and place seam side down in a casserole dish. Sprinkle more bacon and cheese over top of the burritos and bake. (See directions in the recipe card at the bottom of this post for the temperature and time.)

Enjoy them while they're hot! They are so easy to make, and I love that they are a healthy breakfast that my kids love. It's a great way to start the day. If you want to change it up a little and pack an extra punch of flavor try adding this homemade keto enchilada sauce on them!

Meal prepping? Keep reading to see how to reheat your burritos from the fridge or freezer for this easy low carb breakfast recipe.

HOW TO ROLL (OR WRAP) A BREAKFAST BURRITO

Rolling a burrito is not hard to do; it just needs to be tight enough, so the filling does not fall out when you eat it. In this egg and bacon burrito casserole, I did not tuck the ends in, but you will want to do this if you plan on eating the burrito with your hands.

Step 1: Place the filling (eggs, meat, cheese, veggies) in the center of your burrito.

Step 2: If making a hand-held burrito, fold the left and right sides of the burrito inward, slightly overlapping the filling. If making a burrito casserole as I did in this recipe, you do not need to fold the sides in since you will be eating these with a fork and knife.

Step 3: Then start to roll by tucking the bottom of the tortilla underneath the filling and, while keeping the sides folded inward, roll until nice and tight.

Low Carb Keto Chicken Enchiladas

Low carb and keto chicken enchiladas makes for a yummy Mexican inspired dinner no one will even know is low carb. The keto enchiladas with low carb tortillas lets you enjoy enchiladas when you're on a keto diet.

Ingredients

• 2 lb chicken, cubed

•

• 1-2 Tbsp olive oil

•

• 1 cup onion, diced

-
- 1 4oz can of green chilis, drained
-
- 1 tsp cumin
-
- 1/2 tsp chili powder
-
- 1 jar enchilada sauce
-

- 8 Mission Carb Balance tortillas

-

- 2 cups colby jack cheese, shredded

-

- Non-stick cooking spray

Instructions

Preheat the oven to 350F.

Cook the Chicken

In a large skillet over medium-high heat, heat the olive oil in the pan. Cook the onions for 3-4 minutes until the onion starts to soften.

Add the bite-sized chicken pieces, cumin, and chili powder and cook until the pieces are white on the outside. The chicken won't be cooked all the way through at this point, but will finish cooking in the oven. Stir in the drained green chilis.

Feel free to substitute roasted chicken or another type of shredded chicken you might have on hand. Making low carb enchiladas makes perfect use for leftover shredded chicken!

Assemble the Keto Enchilada in Red Sauce

Spray a 9x13" pan with non-stick cooking spray.

Add a large spoonful of enchilada sauce to each tortilla

and spread the sauce on one side of the tortilla.

Add chicken down the center of the tortilla, which will

be about 1/2 cup of chicken.

Sprinkle with a generous sprinkle of cheese.

Roll the tortillas up and place in the baking dish either

seam side up or seam side down.

Pour the remaining enchilada sauce over the top of the keto chicken enchiladas.

Sprinkle the rest of the cheese over the top of the low carb enchiladas recipe.

Bake and Serve

Bake for 15-20 minutes until cooked through and the cheese is melted.

Garnish with cilantro if desired, and serve with sour cream, avocado, salsa, or chives on the side.

Makes 8 servings. Enjoy!

Chipotle Chicken Fajita Bowls (Whole30, Paleo, Keto, Easy Meal Prep)

This recipe for Chipotle Chicken Fajita Bowls is perfect for your next meal prep session. This dish is Paleo, low carb, Whole30 compliant and super tasty! It works for an easy weeknight meal or for quick and easy meal prep lunches.

Ingredients

For The Chicken

• 1–1.5 lbs chicken breast

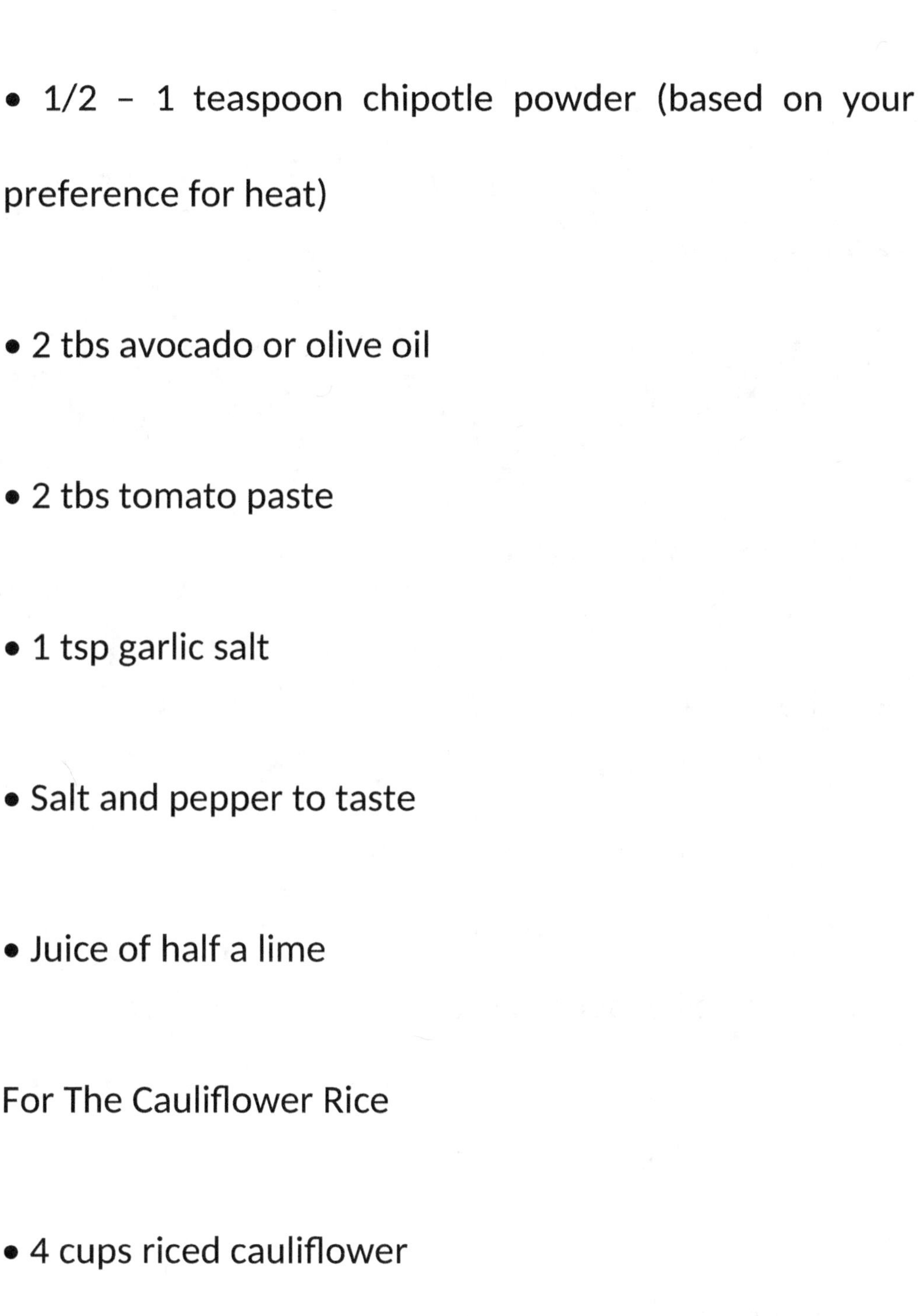

- 1/2 – 1 teaspoon chipotle powder (based on your preference for heat)

- 2 tbs avocado or olive oil

- 2 tbs tomato paste

- 1 tsp garlic salt

- Salt and pepper to taste

- Juice of half a lime

For The Cauliflower Rice

- 4 cups riced cauliflower

- ¼ cup chopped chilantro

- Juice of 1 lime

- 1 tsp garlic salt

- Salt and Pepper to taste

For the Fajita Veggies

- 1 red bell pepper, sliced

- 1 green bell pepper, sliced

- 1 yellow bell pepper, sliced

- 1 orange bell pepper, sliced

- 1 white onion, sliced

- 1 tbs avocado or olive oil

- 1 tsp garlic salt

- 1 tsp cumin

Instructions

. Mix ingredients for chicken marinade (oil, lime juice, chipotle powder, garlic salt, tomato paste) in a small bowl

. Pat chicken breasts dry with a paper towel and place in a freezer bag with marinade and massage bag to coat chicken. Set aside.

. Warm a pan on medium high heat and spray with cooking spray (I use Chosen Foods Avocado Oil Spray

. Add in riced cauliflower, garlic salt, salt and pepper to taste and sauté until cauliflower is tender (about 5-7 minutes).

. Mix cauliflower with lime juice and chopped cilantro in a bowl and set aside

. Keeping pan on medium high heat, add 1 tbs oil and sliced onions. Sauté for about 1-2 minutes

. Add sliced bell peppers , garlic salt and cumin to pan and sauté until veggies are tender but crisp (about 4-5 minutes). Set aside.

. Add additional oil to pan if needed and cook chicken for 4-5 minutes per side (depending on thickness) or until no longer pink

. Assemble bowls with chicken, cauliflower rice and fajita vegetables

. Garnish with lime, cilantro and avocado if desired.

Skinny Meatloaf Muffins with Barbecue Sauce

Prep Time: 15 minutes

Bake Time: 40 minutes

Ingredients for Meatloaf Muffins:

1 package (~1.25 pounds) 99% fat-free ground turkey breast

1 slice whole-wheat or multigrain bread (I used Milton's Multi-Grain) or ½ cup store bought bread crumbs

1 cup onions, finely diced

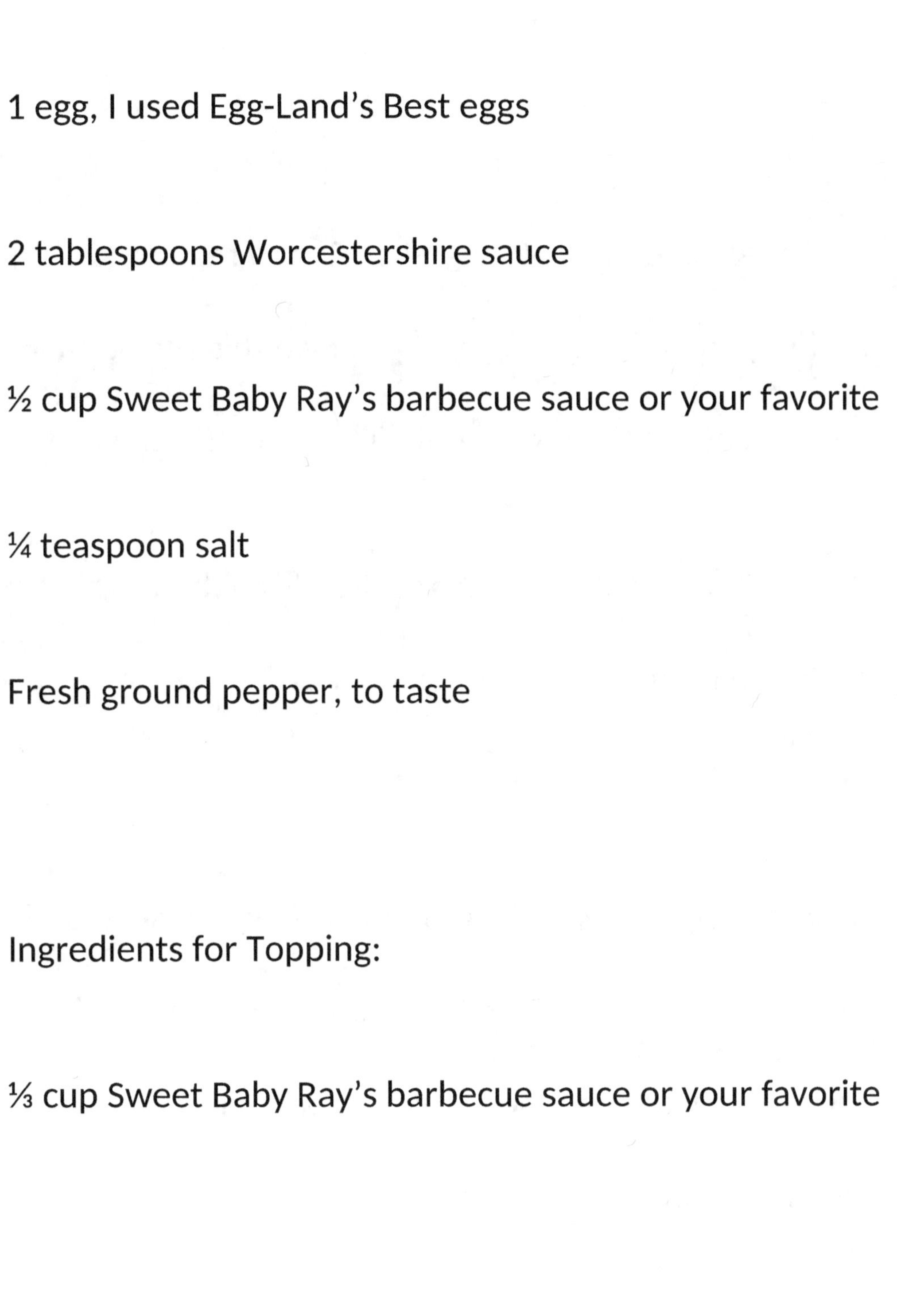

1 egg, I used Egg-Land's Best eggs

2 tablespoons Worcestershire sauce

½ cup Sweet Baby Ray's barbecue sauce or your favorite

¼ teaspoon salt

Fresh ground pepper, to taste

Ingredients for Topping:

⅓ cup Sweet Baby Ray's barbecue sauce or your favorite

Instructions

1. Preheat oven to 350 degrees. Coat a regular (12-cup) muffin pan with cooking spray. Since this recipe makes 9 meatloaf muffins, you'll only fill 9, not 12. Set aside.

2. To make bread crumbs: Toast 1 slice whole-wheat or multi-grain bread. Place in blender and pulse until made into crumbs.

3. In a large bowl, add ground turkey, bread crumbs, onions, egg, Worcestershire sauce, ½ cup barbecue sauce, salt and pepper. Using your hands or a large spoon, thoroughly mix together until well blended.

4. Add meatloaf mixture to the 9 muffin cups, flattening out the tops. Top each meatloaf muffin with ¾ tablespoon barbecue sauce and spread evenly over top.

5. Bake for 40 minutes. Run a knife around each muffin to loosen it from pan. Remove to a serving plate.

Makes 9 meatloaf muffins (1-2 muffins per serving)